J.N.V TO WORLD

An unfinished journey
CHUNCHUN MAHTHA

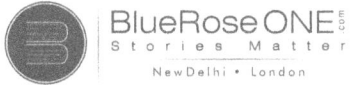

BLUEROSE PUBLISHERS
India | U.K.

Copyright © Chunchun Mahtha 2024

All rights reserved by author. No part of this publication may be reproduced, stored in a retrieval system or transmitted in any form or by any means, electronic, mechanical, photocopying, recording or otherwise, without the prior permission of the author. Although every precaution has been taken to verify the accuracy of the information contained herein, the publisher assumes no responsibility for any errors or omissions. No liability is assumed for damages that may result from the use of information contained within.

BlueRose Publishers takes no responsibility for any damages, losses, or liabilities that may arise from the use or misuse of the information, products, or services provided in this publication.

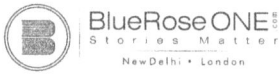

For permissions requests or inquiries regarding this publication, please contact:

BLUEROSE PUBLISHERS
www.BlueRoseONE.com
info@bluerosepublishers.com
+91 8882 898 898
+4407342408967

ISBN: 978-93-5819-886-7

Cover design: Shivani
Typesetting: Sagar

First Edition: July 2024

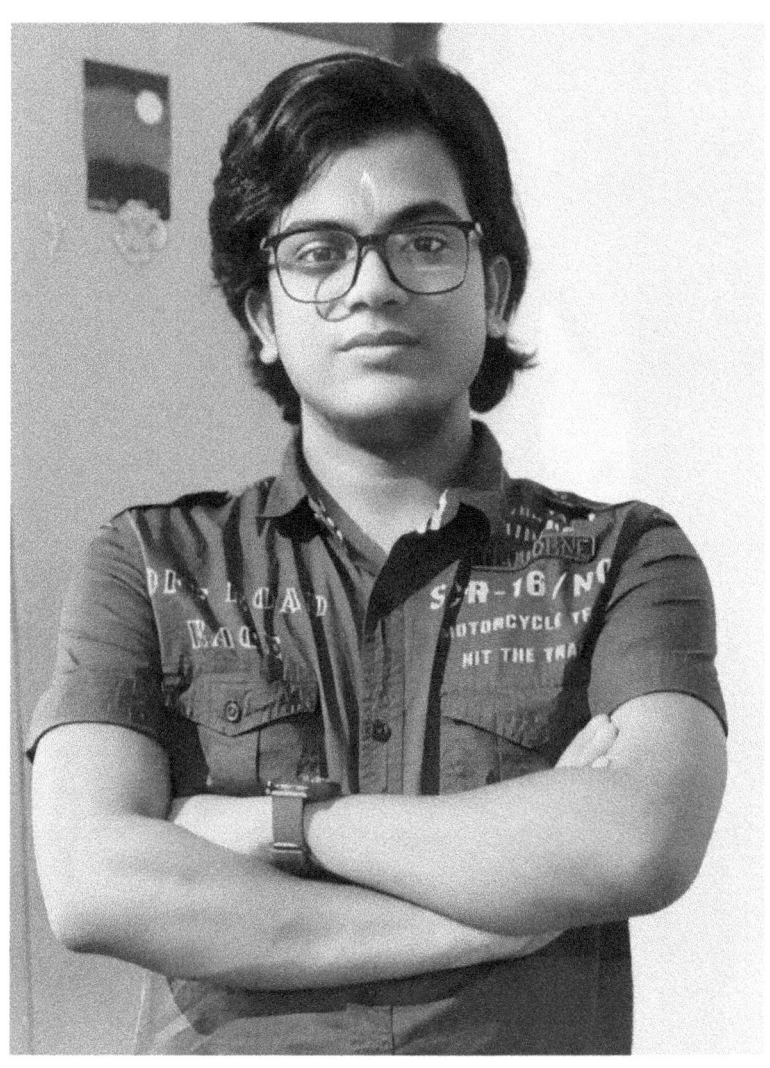

Life starts with struggle and ends with joy

Life begins in misery and ends in death, but determination transforms it. Life commences in struggle and concludes in joy.

There was no respect in the society, Poverty made fun of him a lot because his father was a rickshaw puller. He created such a history that could give a new feeling to millions like himself: that the poor have got the opportunity to be richer than the rich, to earn more respect than what they have made fun of. After all, no one helped him but wonder, how exactly did he manage to do it? The mere thought of his success seemed unimaginable to everyone. Not a single person held any glimmer of hope. Yet, it was solely the influential figures in his life – his parents, brother, sympathizer, and understanding sister who bestowed upon him the unwavering determination and fortitude to pursue his cherished dream.

The earthen house, decorated with rags and shining with lamps, had to be entered with the head down like a temple. Seeing this, everyone would comment on how small the house was, like cows and goats lived there. However, the parents would say that home is like a temple. They didn't want their child to feel poor because his father didn't have a good home, Bank balance, so they always tried to provide satisfaction by speaking positively. But this boy was not one of those who just listened; he was one of the doers. He wanted to have the spirit to give a befitting reply to those who made fun of him. What did he do? How did he do it or not?

Parents and their five children were lying on beds. Mr J was saying to the elder sons that kittu had to enrol tomorrow. kittu became very happy upon hearing that he would go to school. His parents also became happy seeing that he was happy instead of being afraid. Upon hearing the school name, the other children cried, but he was smiling a lot.

A new chapter is about to be written to forge a fresh era of historical significance. Early in the morning, his mother got ready. Then she went to worship and after returning, she woke up her dearest son, Nandlal. She saw that he was already ready, so she asked when he had gotten ready. He said that he got up when she had gone to worship, and immediately went to wash up and take a bath. Hearing all this, tears came to his mother's eyes. So Kittu asked his mother why she was crying, and he lovingly said he knew it was because of happiness. His mother replied, 'Yes, but it was not true.' While she was thinking that, kittu said, 'Maa,' and she came out of her deep thoughts. At that time, her eyes fell on his clothes. She said with a smile, 'Oh Nandlal, come, let me prepare you a little better and apply oil on your head.' She dressed him properly and combed his hair like an innocent child. She applied kajal to his eyes and a tika of kajal on his forehead and behind his ear so that no one could cast an evil eye on her child. Then she applied Navratna powder while preparing Kittu. She said, 'Oh God, please take care of my son.'

Kittu and his mother excitedly awaited the arrival of Mr. Goran J, Kittu's father, who left early in the morning to drive a rickshaw, ensuring that they had everything they needed at home. Mr. Goran J arrived right on time. Bringing joy to Kittu who exclaimed, 'Papa is here, Mom! Let's give him food and head to school together, the three of us.' With enthusiasm, Punam D., Kittu's Mom , quickly sliced an onion. They had two leftover breads from the previous night, and one was lovingly given to Kittu's father. She generously shared more than half of the bread with her son enjoying the remaining portion herself. After the satisfying meal, Kittu cheerfully hopped onto the rickshaw, followed by his mother. As they set off, he couldn't contain his excitement and cheerfully urged his father, 'Papa, let's go quickly!' With a smile, his father happily drove them to school.

Principal chamber, GKMS school

He had the privilege of standing before the esteemed principal, while his parents anxiously sat beside him. Inquisitive by nature, Mr. KN Jha(principal) directed a series of compelling questions towards Kittu.

Mr. KN Jha inquires, 'What's your name?'

Kittu confidently responds, 'My name is Kittu Kumar, although my mother affectionately refers to me as Nandlal.'

Curious, Mr. KN Jha further asks, 'And what is your father's name?'

Kittu promptly replies, 'My father's name is Mr. Goran J, but my mother respectfully addresses him as 'ji.'

With a warm smile, Mr. KN Jha inquires, 'Where is your home, young one?'

Without hesitation, Kittu proudly states, 'My home resides in the tender embrace of my mother, Mrs. Punam D.' As Punam D. Hears these words, her eyes glisten brightly like shining pearls. The principal happily announced that he now has to answer two questions.

1st question – How much is two -two? Kittu replied, saying Principal Ji must be twenty-two.

The principal asked, 'How will it happen?' Please describe a little. At that time, his parents started looking at him. Then Kittu replied that if you asked how much two plus two would be, then it would have been four. You did not mention anything about addition, subtraction, multiplication, or division. That's why two -two equals twenty-two.

The principal was impressed by this and said, 'What a wonderful description such a small child has given.' Kittu's parents were happy to hear that.

2nd question: As the child grows up, his clothes become smaller. Is it correct?

Kittu replied, saying no, completely wrong. When the child grows up, the child's height is increasing. That's why the clothes seem small to us. While we grow up, the clothes do not become small.

After observing these remarkable abilities, Mr. KN Jha confidently approached Kittu's parents, expressing that their child demonstrates exceptional intellect and is well-suited for enrolment in the 2nd class.

The parents, elated by this news, received it with joy, and swiftly completed Kittu's enrolment process. Kittu was embraced by his mother, who subsequently returned home alongside both of them, inciting an uproar throughout the entire vicinity due to Goran J's son's exceptional performance at school. Despite their intent to enrol him in the first class, the principal himself decided to place him in the second class. This resulted in a mix of admiration and envy among the onlookers. Many individuals were on the verge of becoming envious, thus attributing the principal's decision to Goran J's compassionate nature and some people were saying that his father was transporting the principal's daughter to school, which is why Kittu got admission in 2nd class. Nevertheless, Mr. Goran J's family members were elated.

This is not even the dawn of a new era. Kittu's parents were anxiously discussing late into the night while seated on the rickshaw. Mrs. J expressed her concern, stating that tomorrow Kittu would be going to school. She worriedly questioned how he would obtain the necessary pencil and slate because they had no money.

Mrs. J acknowledged that Mr. J had been preoccupied with Kittu's enrolment, preventing him from going to work that day.

In response, Mr J reassured her, saying, 'Do not fret. I will make the necessary arrangements in the morning.'

Affirming her faith in him, Mrs. J replied, 'Of course, I know you will handle it.'

#First day of school #

Early in the morning, Mr. J anxiously rushed to TK Singh, his friend and a lender. Mrs. J's worries intensified as she noticed the distress on her husband's face, confirming her suspicions that he had failed to borrow the money. Desperate for answers, Mrs. J inquired about the turn of events.

With a heavy heart, Mr. J divulged that he had requested financial assistance from TK Singh, who initially agreed to provide it. However, as he handed over the money, the lender questioned the urgency, forcing Mr. J to explain the situation. After explaining , unexpectedly, the lender began making excuses, claiming to be preoccupied and unable to fulfil his promise.

Touched by disillusionment, Mrs. J astutely grasped the bitter truth that nobody would extend a helping hand if their child were to pursue an education. Immediately, Mr. J declared his intention to drive the rickshaw and purchase a pencil and slate for his son. For a brief moment, there was silence as his wife contemplated his decision. Eventually, she resolutely

Offered to sell her gold nose pin, explaining that she no longer wore it. Mr. J Swiftly interjected, questioning the possibility of selling such a significant Symbol of their marriage. Undeterred, she emphasized that if Kittu focused on His studies, they would acquire plenty of nose pin. Overwhelmed by this unwavering Support, tears welled up in Mr. J's eyes. Deeply moved, he decided to mortgage her gold nose pin in order to acquire the necessary funds for the pencil and Slate.

Kittu wore his elder brother's school uniform. Ashirvad flour packet was used As a bag. Slate, pencil, and a small piece of cloth(to clean the slate) were put in the bag.

On their way to school, his elders kindly Purchased Haldiram, Munch, and a Parle-G biscuit, which they lovingly handed over to Kittu. The sight of this thoughtful gesture filled Kittu's heart with immense joy and happiness.

* A Glimpse of Success *

The president of the USA called the prime minister of India.

President of the USA: We need 'Akshat!.

PM of India: I will inform you some time later.

After hanging up the call, the PM asked his PA, Where is he?"

PA patiently answered, 'Sir, currently he is in japan.

PM: How long will he take time in Japan?

PA, with a little fear: sir, I am not sure.

He exhibited a diminutive physical stature, yet his actions greatly surpassed Those of the older individuals. Many children were standing in long queues and a very tall blond man with a stick was jokingly ordering the children to stand straight in the queue. Seven or eight girls were standing in front of all the pupils with braids tied, and teachers were standing next to them. One of the teachers was a fat, pot-bellied man with a sandalwood tilak on his forehead.

Saying to start the prayer. Seeing all this, Kittu was feeling very strange. He himself could not understand whether he was feeling good or bad, but he was definitely feeling that he..

After the prayer ,all the students went to their respective classes. In Second grade, some children were gossiping among themselves that one boy gave all the answers and the principal himself praised him. Then one child said excitedly, 'look at the one who sat in front, the one with the bag of Ashirvad Flour packet.' Then all the students began to look at him. Kittu turned back after hearing that and seeing everyone, a charming smile came on his face.

A boy asked Kittu what his name was, and he replied, wait for a While, the teacher would ask then listen.' Immediately, the teacher came and all The children stood up and addressed her, 'Good morning, teacher, the whole Class echoed. She also addressed and said, 'Good morning to the future of the Great nation.

She was the teacher of moral education. She started telling a story about a boy who did not feel like going to school. Whenever it was time to go to school, he would make excuses that he had a headache or stomach ache so his father would take him to the doctor. As soon as he reached the doctor, he would immediately say that he was fine. On the first day, his father laughed after hearing that. He kept doing it like that for two to three days when actually one day his head was hurting. He said that his head was hurting and started crying. When his father came upstairs and saw him, they thought that again he was making an excuse and sent him to school. The child died on the way to school. When his post-mortem was done, it was found in the investigation that he died due to internal bleeding in the head. Then his father wondered how this happened, he went home and checked the camera recording and saw that when he was getting ready to go to school, he slipped and his head hit the floor, and he got hurt internally, and he was normal from outside it seems. And then he started screaming right there, his father was waiting for him. When it was getting late downstairs, his father went upstairs to see him and saw that he was shouting that his head was hurting, but his father felt that like every time, that time also he was pretending.

Seeing this camera recording videos his father started crying a lot and started repenting. So the teacher taught them that we should not lie, even a lie can prove to be dangerous for life.

Madam quizzed the students to see if they were able to grasp the concept. And to her delight, every single pupil chimed in unison, 'yes, teacher.' Intriguingly, right after that, a curious child bravely rose from their seat and inquired, 'Is there a lie out there that surpasses even the grandeur of life? Would someone actually face losing their life for daring to utter such a falsehood?' The teacher became silent for a few moments and then she asked the boy what he wanted to say.

The boy explained that life is more precious than a lie. In the story, his father thought he was lying, so he didn't pay any attention. This means he considered the lie to be bigger. If he considered life to be bigger, his son would have lied a thousand times. Yet they go to the doctor because there is nothing more important than life. After losing his son, they must have known that, which is why they started regretting. Then the boy asked the teacher if he was saying anything wrong. The entire class fell into a peaceful hush.

A warm smile graced the teacher's face as they kindly suggested to the students, 'Let's all show our appreciation by giving a big round of applause for that extraordinary boy. The teacher asked the boy what his name was. The boy answered that his name is Kittu Kumar and his mother called him Nandlal. The teacher said that she too learned a new thing, and happily blessed him, saying that he would go far ahead in life. There was a discussion in the school that, upon hearing Kittu's answer, everyone became silent.

Kittu came home and said everything about his first day of school. His mother became extremely happy upon hearing this.

To be committed, one morning, while Mrs. J was standing in the street, Mrs. Monica (Kittu's aunt) was coming after dropping her kids off at a private school. Mrs. S. Ramani (Kittu's neighbour) asked Mrs. Monica where she was coming from. She replied in a mocking tone that she had come after leaving her children in a government school with great teachers, and they both started laughing.

While Kittu's cousins studied in reputed private schools, Mrs. Monica was taunting Mrs. J because Punam D's sons studied in a government school. She got very Upset hearing this and cursed herself. Wondering why she was poor'?

When Kittu came back from school and saw his mother in sorrow, then he asked his mother, "What happened, maa?" She didn't say anything, Then again, he asked, "What happened to you? Please share with me.'

Mrs J replied that he had to study a lot. Kittu said that yes, he would . Again, Kittu asked, What Happened?" Then his mother mentioned the morning incident. Knowing that, Kittu became enraged. He felt that some new power was coming into him.

Then he promised his mother that he would study harder than anyone has ever done or thought of. Hearing all this, his mother hugged him and said, 'It is my blessing. At a young age, he possessed such immense ambition that he believed he could truly make a difference in the world, and he always motivated others to join him in striving for greatness. He would often proclaim, no matter what obstacles come our way, remember that whatever is meant to Be will align with God's will., and God also shares the same desires as Kittu."

The principal announced that two students have successfully passed the JNV Entrance exam and would pursue further studies JNV. They would receive free provisions including food, accommodation, stationery, Textbooks, school Uniforms, footwear, and education. It is observed that students who study from JNV perform exceptionally well in life and achieve great success. This information triggered Kittu's recollection of his mother's words, which affirmed his potential for a prosperous future. Consequently, he became determined to explore the opportunities offered by JNV and began inquiries regarding admission procedures and preparation strategies.

Kittu diligently sought guidance from his teachers on how to excel in the exam, garnering immense respect and admiration from all. Remarkably, among his teachers, Mrs. Punam Sharma held a special place in her heart for him, coincidentally sharing the same name as Kittu's mother. It was Mrs. Sharma who advised him to purchase a comprehensive book and emphasized the necessity of seeking additional tuition for thorough preparation.

Now Kittu was in third grade. All the pupils in the class were taking tuition except one or two. Kittu was one of them. He studied on his own and used to practice at home whatever was taught in school. Being a government school, not much was taught. There were only one or two teachers who taught sincerely, the rest just came to break the school chairs. It seemed as if they all came to complete the unfinished household work like knitting sweaters, etc., and not to impart education.

He started pondering on the daunting task of figuring out a way to attend JNV amidst this predicament. The growing concern that his cousin, attending a prestigious private school and receiving additional tutoring, added to his worries. Helpless Kittu, who lacked the privilege of attending renowned schools or having tutoring, felt extremely dejected whenever he struggled to grasp anything. What course of action should he take now? With great distress. He confided in his mother and shared everything. After Thoughtful deliberation, his mother enthusiastically shared the news that his maternal grandfather, a highly educated police officer, would be his mentor. The tremendous joy that lit up his face upon hearing that he would also receive tuition was truly heart-warming. Blessed with the opportunity to further his education, he eagerly anticipated making the most of every moment.

First day of tuition

He arose early in the morning and proceeded to prepare himself independently. In proceeding with these morning tasks, the time elapsed to 9 o'clock. Thereafter, he consumed the remnants of rice from the previous night's meal before making his way to school, where he remained until 10 am. During the evening, he typically concluded his schooling at 4pm; however, due to the considerable distance, he would not return until 5 pm. As soon as he arrived back, he would Promptly visit his maternal grandfather's residence to engage in focused studying while still attired in his school uniform, as his grandfather's abode was situated nearby.

He memorized tables up to twenty, counting up to a hundred in two days and learned to read English literature. Mr. RK (Kittu's maternal Grandfather) said that his learning speed was too fast. He used to learn everything very quickly. But what would be the use of studying for one or two Years? In the end, he would only drive a rickshaw. Kittu got disappointed after hearing that.

A Glimpse of Success

The prime minister called back the president of the USA.

PM : We are sorry to say that Akshat is busy right now; he will only be able to go afterFour to five months. President of the USA: If you will try, he can come soon. There are a lot of problems happening in the USA;his arrival is very urgent

PM : I will try.

Upon the completion of his tuition, Kittu returned to his abode appearing rather despondent. Noticing his sombre countenance, his mother inquired about the cause of his distress. However, Kittu chose to withhold any mention of Nana ji, as he wished to spare his mother from disappointment.

One day, something happened. After his school day had ended, he promptly proceeded to Nana ji's residence to engage in studying without taking a moment's respite at home. Despite experiencing hunger pangs, Kittu remained committed to his academic pursuits and departed without partaking in any sustenance. After studying tuition, Kittu munched on the chapatti that Nani ji had saved for Nana ji. When Nana ji caught him in the act, he got mad at Kittu. It made Kittu feel super bummed since he had only eaten a piece of bread, not stolen anything. Why did Nana ji react like that? And once again, Kittu didn't utter a word to his mom.

At night, Kittu was like, 'Yo mom, why is everyone always telling me not to study? Like, why do they think I can only drive a rickshaw?'

His mom, on the real, used to tell him that it was all for Nandlal's good, but Kittu would get all annoyed and upset. So then his mom was like, 'If you feel bummed out, then you gotta study even harder.' And Kittu was like, 'Yeah, I do feel bummed out.' So his mom straight up told him to keep on studying and not stop. He expressed his intention to dedicate increased effort towards his studies henceforth. Subsequently, following the evening meal, all individuals retired for the night. With firm conviction, she explicitly emphasized that he ought not to perceive himself as inferior to others. Her Intention was to shield him from awareness of the derogatory remarks that Circled due to his father's profession as a rickshaw puller.

In childhood, other Children used to have so much fun. They used to play as soon as the evening fell but he neither had any means to have fun nor did he have time to play. He was obsessed with studies and going to Navodaya. It's been four months since he studied tuition, and he learned almost everything, which was enough to Prepare for JNV entrance exam. Now he wanted to start his preparation, for this he needed a book and a teacher who taught him sincerely.

Kittu told his mother that he wanted to prepare for JNV and needed a book for that. His mother asked how much money it would cost. Already, Kittu had Asked the price of the book from book sellers, 200rs. His mother said that she would give the money by Sunday. A big challenge arose for Mrs J as to how She would arrange the money for the book.", Now her mother began fretting about the source of such a substantial amount of money. Her husband used to barely make seventy to eighty rupees a day, which was far from sufficient to cover the expenses of the household. An idea came to her mind that she would Send her three sons (S.K, J.K, and Kittu) to their maternal grandfather's home. And the younger daughter (G.k) to her aunt's home. If the youngest one (Anuj) Who only drinks mother's milk, she would keep him with herself She would then fast for two days and tell her husband that he should eat outside because She would not be cooking at home for two days. Mrs J did the same and did not spend anything for two days (Friday and Saturday).In this way, she was able to save Rs. 180. Kittu's mother gave him the money on Sunday evening and told him to tell the bookshop owner that he would pay back the 20 Rs that he owed. Even after making so many sacrifices, she was only able to save 180 rupees. Now she understood that the money could be needed at any time for Kittu's studies, and she also knew that there would be no immediate arrangements or anyone to help. There were household expenses and no money could be saved. Her husband believed that no matter what happened, there should never be any shortage of food. All the money they earned was spent on providing food and nothing was saved. So Mrs. J thought that from now on she would reduce expenses and save money for studies. As soon as Kittu got the money, he ran to the book seller and asked if the book could cost only Rs. 180, even though he knew the book's price.Mr. MK (the book shop owner) said that it would not be that much. Kittu did not mention what his mother had said because he felt that when the shopkeeper heard it, Mr. MK would not agree. An idea came to his mind that he would clean the shop for a month and ask some of his school friends to buy books only from MK shop. He told the shopkeeper that he would bring more customers to the shop and clean it every morning for a month. Mr.MK thought about it for a while and then asked Kittu if he was up for the task. Kittu replied confidently, 'Sure, I woudl !' and Mr . MK handed over the book for Rs. 180. Grabbing the book, he rushed home.

The moment Mrs. J caught sight of the book, she treated it like royalty and blessed her son, predicting his success on the exam. Kittu then spilled the beans to his mom, revealing that he had only charged 180 rupees for the book. His mother was overjoyed upon hearing this, but Kittu didn't offer any further explanation" When Papa got back home around 9 pm, He spotted Kittu engrossed in a book and thought it was pretty cool.

Suddenly, Papa's eyes locked onto the book and he asked where he got it from, Without hesitation, Mrs. J quickly chimed in, saying that the teacher had handed it to him for reading This left Kittu wondering why mom fibbed.

Once they Finished dinner, Mrs. J had a heart-to-heart with Kittu, explaining that Papa was Already super stressed about his older brother's health and she didn't want to burden him further. If she had told the truth. It would have only caused him more worry. Don't worry, though, she promised to tell him later. Mrs. J kindly Urged Kittu to focus on his studies, assuring him that he has the support of his Mother.

Every single day, with enthusiasm bubbling inside him, Kittu would Joyfully rise before the crack of dawn to meticulously clean the outside of the Shop, ensuring it sparkled without a hint of imperfection. Once his task was Completed, he would eagerly head back home and readily surrender to sweet Slumber, embracing his mother's schedule as his own.

On Friday, October 10, 2003. Mrs. J woke up Nandlal from his sleep and told him to brush his teeth and eat the rice left from the night. She then instructed him to study for some time before going to school. He followed her instructions and went to school Where he informed his classmates that the JNV entrance exam would be held in February 2006. If they started preparing from that moment, it would ensure that All of them would pass. Some children agreed while others paid no attention. The class consisted of 250 students, out of which 15 children were ready to Start preparing from that point on. The child became very curious and asked Kittu how they should prepare. In response, Kittu enthusiastically suggested that they should buy a book and take tuition. This answer intrigued all the boys who eagerly asked Kittu where they could get the book. With a mischievous grin, Kittu proposed that they should all visit his house in the evening, each bringing 200 rupees. After school ended, the children excitedly went to their respective homes, and astonishingly, 10 of them managed to gather the money and arrive at Kittu's house. With utmost secrecy, Kittu led them all to MK's shop, without Mrs. J knowing. In the evening, an unprecedented number of pupils gathered at MK's establishment, leaving him astounded by the sheer volume of children present, given the educational limitations prevailing in the locality. Kittu proudly declared that he had brought along his comrades, each keen on acquiring JNV books. This revelation stirred MK's curiosity, pondering over the profound transformation of Kittu who had voiced a similar intention only a few days prior, yet managed to entice such a considerable group of young learners in such a short span of time. Subsequently, every child completed their purchases before departing for their respective homes. But Kittu stayed there, and all the children went home.

'MK was all like, Dude, you're an awesome boy! How can I get everyone to buy my book? And how did you convince the children to buy books?' Kittu was like, 'MK uncle, if your heart's in the right place, the whole universe will have your back.' Man, Mr. MK was blown away by that deep stuff coming from such a little dude. MK assured Kittu he'd totally achieve greatness one day. They chatted a bit more before heading home.

"17 Oct, Thursday: when Mrs. Got up in the morning to urinate, she did not see Nandlal on the bed. So she Went out to look, but Kittu was nowhere to be found. She was completely frightened and unable to understand what to do next. Then a woman (datvan Seller) appeared with a twig of Neem, Datun, on her head. She was passing by (had to go to the market before sunrise to sell Datun).

Mrs. J asked the woman If she had seen a child, and she said yes. Mrs. J quickly asked where, and the Woman replied towards the bookshop.

Poonam D went running; the shop was Near the house, and she saw that her Nandlal was sweeping. Upon seeing Kittu Sweeping, blood streamed from Mrs J's eyes instead of tears. Even in the Absence of an earthquake, she sensed the ground trembling beneath her feet. With a sense of concern, she cried out, 'What are you doing? Startled.

Kittu turned around and caught sight of his mother, which filled him with fear. However, upon seeing tears streaming down her face, he hurried over to her Side. She started crying a lot and asked Kittu why the shopkeeper had told him to do the work because he had not given his 20 rupees. She wondered how he dared to say to Nandlal to broom and started crying completely. Kittu also Started crying along with her and said, Mom, don't cry. Please don't cry.'

Seeing Kittu crying, Mrs. J calms herself down and then asks, "Why were you Sweeping? Tell me everything?

Then Kittu told the whole matter that the shopkeeper had not told him to work.

He was sweeping as he wished so that he would not have to give Rs. 20 to his mother. Then his mother said that she would have given it. Kittu said that he Knew how his mother had given him the money. He did not want to trouble his mother even more, so he thought of doing it himself. His mother was completely shocked to hear all this and told Kittu that he had shown so much wisdom at such a young age. She said that he would bring glory to his parents in the whole world. After saying this, Mrs. J tried to carry him in her lap. Nandlal told his mother that he had grown up and how could she bear his weight. She smiled and said, 'Son, a mother can do anything for her son. When a child is in the mother's womb, it doesn't have weight for a mother, but it weighs more than anything else in the world.' She forcefully took him in her lap and started towards home. He understood something, but the rest went out of his mind. On the way, he told his mother that he used to understand everything about others at once but couldn't understand his mother's statement. So he asked, 'Why, mom?' His mother said that she is a mother. A mother understands everything her sons say without speaking, but the sons do not understand. Even after saying it, the sons ignore it. If the sons start understanding, then all the problems of the parents will end. Kittu, once again, could not understand what she was trying to say. However, he asked if he understood, all of his mother's problems would end. Then she said, 'Yes, Nandlal.' He then said that from now on, he would try to understand everything. His mother smiled, and they both reached home. After coming home, he slept, but his mother's worry persisted as she continued to believe that her son was sleeping. The image of that scene relentlessly replayed in her mind, causing her to anxiously contemplate finding ways to save money. After a duration of 2 hours, Kittu was roused from his slumber by his mother. In the process of rising, he expressed his reluctance to attend school on that particular day. In response, his mother calmly reassured him, "That is not an issue, but Please make yourself prepared." After getting ready, he thought that Durga Puja was over on the 5th of October and Diwali was coming up real quick on The 25th. So, he told his mom, 'Hey Mom, Sir told me that everyone has a great Time and lots of fun during these celebrations.' Then, he asked if both his mom and dad wouldn't join in on the fun. He couldn't understand why his parents didn't want to celebrate. His mom fell silent after that. After a few seconds she said, 'What happened, Babu? Papa brings clothes and Sweets for everyone.' Kittu said that he was not talking about himself or his Brothers and sisters; he was talking about mom and dad. He asked why Papa Has not bought even a single new clothes, and if he buys them for you then you ask him to return them and have never seen Papa taking them. Why do both of You get upset during the festival? Everyone is so happy on the occasion of puja, Why not both of you? Mother playfully brushed off the matter, suggesting that He was merely staying at home to bring a little mischief into his mother's life.

She added with a cheerful laugh that she would send him to school soon enough. Inquisitive as ever, Kittu pressed on, asking for more information. With a smile, she replied, 'Son, when you grow up, you will understand.'

When Mr. J arrived at 10 o'clock, he noticed that Kittu was at home and kindly Inquired with his mother about why our son didn't go to school. She explained that he simply didn't feel like going today. Mr. J then smiled and jokingly asked if he bombarded her with questions or not. Mrs. J replied, 'Of course he did! How could he resist? Could you even imagine?' this led to hearty laughter between the two of them. Hearing some giggles, Kittu also arrived and casually asked what Papa and Mummy were chatting and giggling about. They replied that they were just showering praises on him. Then Kittu playfully chimed in, 'Who's getting all this love?' and cutely threatened, 'Spill the beans, or I might just burst into tears.' That got both of them laughing, and of course, Kittu couldn't resist joining in too. Mr. J joyfully purchased onions from the shop along with a delightful chocolate worth 0.50 rupees. With great elation, they combined the bread, onion, and water, relishing every bite of their meal. Once finished, Mr. J generously gifted a chocolate to Kittu, who cheerfully proceeded to divide it into three pieces. One piece went to his grateful father, another to his appreciative mother, and he kept the remaining one for himself. Witnessing this considerate act, his parents were filled with immense joy.

A glimpse of ruling the world

In The Witwatersrand Basin (South Africa)

Mnr. Sikandar: Meneer, ons sal meer belegging vereis.
Die G: Hoekom?

Mnr. Sikandar: Meneer, ons besigheid gaan baie goed, en as ons wil voortgaan, as ons die hele wêreld wil regeer, behoort al die goud ons te wees.

Die G: Goed.

They spent half an hour talking. After that, Mr. J went to drive the Rickshaw, and Mrs. J started cooking while Kittu helped his mother. In the Evening, he also went with his mother to fetch wood. Throughout the day, he Watched his mother to see how much work she did. At night, when Mr. J and Mrs. J were lying on the bed to sleep, Kittu started massaging their legs, then his parents told him to stop. They always blessed him a lot. Then, Kittu said that he was not doing it for blessings but to serve.

The next day, he attended school and noticed that those ten children were engaged in crafting something using the JNV book. Kittu also realized that all Of them were receiving tutorial lessons for JNV. Considering studying Independently, he planned to seek assistance at school whenever he encountered difficulties. Kittu started studying and managed to tackle Reasoning questions independently, although he struggled with mathematics. As A result, he approached his teacher for guidance in school . However, when Kittu sought Clarification on mathematical concepts, the teacher would first review the Question's solution before providing an explanation . Unfortunately, the Teacher's explanations proved inadequate, and by the time he could answer a Single, or at best, two queries, time would run out. In such a manner, he was unable to adequately prepare for his studies, thus expressing his desire to his Mother to seek additional tuition that would enable him to adequately prepare.

He further expressed his inability to achieve the required level of preparedness under the guidance of either Nana ji or within the school. Understanding his Concerns, his mother permitted him to seek tuition, instructing him to identify a suitable tutor. Conveniently, there was a respectable gentleman residing nearby Whose previous students had successfully gained admission into JNV. Hence ,Kittu expressed his interest in studying under this tutor and approached him With his request, which was met with a positive response. They agreed upon fee for tutoring services amounted to Rs 150 per month.

On the 14th of November, he told his mother about the fee. Which was Rs 150. His mother responded affirmatively, stating, 'Very well, devote yourself to your studies.' His teaching hours were from 6pm to 7pm in the evening. Upon commencing his studies on The first day, he offered 5 rupees to Sir after completing his session. At this Point, SK Sharma, the tuition instructor, inquired about Kittu's intentions. Kittu reassured his teacher that he would diligently study every day and make daily payments. Sir advised him against such a practice, suggesting that he pay at the End of the month instead. In response, Kittu explained that his mother had Instructed him to collect 5 rupees each day from his father, a rickshaw driver and give the money to Sir, as she would not be able to provide the full sum of Rs. 150 all at once. Sir understood his domestic situation and said that there Was no problem; he could give it as he wished. Just four days had passed since he started studying when suddenly Sir became ill, and Kittu was given leave for a week. Then his mother kept the money that was left, and when it became 20

Rupees, Kittu asked for the 20 rupees as he had some work. His mother gave it to him without asking anything because she knew that whatever he did, he did It for the good. Kittu approached Mr. MK with 20 rupees and handed them to him.

To MK's astonishment, he questioned why Kittu was giving him money even after he had already swept and assisted with book sales. Intriguingly, Kittu Clarified that MK had placed his trust in him by giving him a book, enabling him to study and be prepared. With that said, Kittu left for home, leaving Mr.MK bewildered and struggling to comprehend his intentions. It turned out that Kittu had also taken on the role of persuading the child to buy books and had Compensated him with money. This left the book seller perplexed, lost in Endless contemplation, God creates strange games that are beyond everyone's Understanding.

In 2003, especially during the months of November and December, someone was laying the foundation of building their empire, while In another corner of the world, the foundation of someone else's empire was about to end.

In India, a person was emerging who was about to make their mark on the entire world, and in Iraq, there was a person whose identity was about to be completely destroyed. Battleground Iraq November 2003.

November was a particularly bloody month for coalition forces in Iraq. Someone was captured on December 13, 2003, and he was subsequently Convicted of crimes against humanity and executed on December 30, 2006.

First time on TV

Kittu's first interview aired on TV due to a scholarship on December 13, 2003, and on December 30, 2006, a new chapter in his life began to build a new Empire. The magnitude of God's theatrical production knows no boundaries; While certain individuals may stumble, others ascend gracefully.

After arriving home, he sat in close proximity to his mother. His mother was aware that he gave the money to the proprietor of the bookshop. She commended his commendable deed and imparted instructions to him to contribute abundantly to society while refraining from taking anything from others. Kittu pledged to abide by his mother counsel, assure Mrs.J of his compliance. As a week passed, Mr. Sharma began to teach. He was astounded by Kittu's rapid grasp of the subject matter. Kittu managed to complete JNV Maths in a mere span of 15 to 20 days. The teacher explained one question, and then Kittu solved all the remaining similar questions himself, completing them very quickly.

On December 8, 2003, a maths competition was organized in which all the government school children from 3rd to 8th grade could participate. Kittu also participated and got the third position in the district, which earned him a scholarship and an interview on December 13th. Kittu's sir and parents were very happy to see him on TV. His reputation spread throughout the district; at such a young age, he was outperforming the elders. He started studying even more, dedicating approximately 13 hours a day to his studies. Mr. Sharma taught him math up to the 8th grade and also had him review JNV. His class teacher even asked him to teach math to the entire class. He became so well-known that almost everyone remembered his name.

Mr. J used to take a young girl named Nidhi to SFS school, who was studying in the fifth grade. She had also heard of Kittu. When Nidhi wanted to meet him. She asked Mr. J. Then, Mr. J said that if her parents allow, he would take her. Nidhi then sought permission from her parents and went to meet Kittu. She talked to him and liked it very much. Nidhi asked Kittu if he would teach her maths. He replied that he would teach her, but after 7 o'clock. Nidhi then said that she would come at 8 o'clock in the night. Despite being In third class, Kittu could teach maths to class eight students. He started teaching her daily. While teaching Nidhi, his math skills improved significantly. Nidhi, who was quite affluent, generously brought him chocolates, biscuits, notebooks, pens, and clothes, gaining a great deal of respect for him. She held a strong desire for Kittu to achieve success in his life as he came from a financially disadvantaged background.

By 2005, Kittu was in the fifth grade while Nidhi was in the seventh grade. Surprisingly, he completed Nidhi's seventh-grade math syllabus as early as October, driven by his anticipation for the upcoming JNV entrance exam. As November arrived, Kittu shifted his focus solely towards his own studies. As soon as Kittu returned from school, he used to go to tuition at 6 o'clock. Then, after coming home, he would eat whatever was available in the house and start studying. Nidhi used to come at 8 pm not for taking tuition,for helping him and ask questions continuously for two hours, as well as take tests of him. As the exam was approaching, sir and Nidhi started giving more time. Sir gave from 6 pm to 8 pm and Nidhi started taking more time for tests, from 8 pm to 11 pm. She also started bringing food from her home for him. Complete preparations had been made and the day was also about to come.

On January 1st, 2006, Nidhi's family had a great day out enjoying themselves. However, she chose to spend the day with Kittu at his home and join in the celebrations. Later, they decided to study together too, making it a productive day. Just before leaving, Nidhi kindly handed a gift to him ,adding a playful remark to only open it once Navodaya is gone. Afterwards, she happily headed back to her own home.

From February 2nd, Nidhi stopped going to school and started helping Kittu throughout the day.On 5th February, Nidhi told Kittu to study at home, and she would go to school and bring the admit card for him.

11th February, Saturday, a day before the exam date. It looked like both Kittu and his mother, along with Nidhi, were preparing for the entrance exams the next day. Nidhi had a plan to visit Kittu's house at 5 a.m. And was even thinking of bringing some delicious bread pakoda along. Her intention was to kindly motivate Kittu to wake up early and study. Unfortunately, when she reached Kittu's house, she realized that his mother had already taken him to study. Nidhi then asked him if there was anything she could help with in their preparation, but he assured her that they were all set. However, Kittu came up with the helpful suggestion that she could create questions from any part of the entire book. Nidhi had come over for the first time so early in the morning.

Out of Mrs. J's kindness, she decided to prepare breakfast for both of them. Mrs. J kindly invited them to have breakfast. In response, Nidhi explained that she had actually brought it for herself and Kittu. With a warm smile, Mrs. J told Nidhi not to bring any for him. In an effort to find a solution, Nidhi suggested that she would enjoy what Mrs. J had prepared, and Mrs. J could have what Nidhi had brought. This idea made Mrs. J smile, and the three of them happily began their breakfast together. During the meal, Nidhi and Mrs. J lovingly fed Kittu, while Mrs. J fed one more bite than Nidhi to Kittu. Overwhelmed with affection, Nidhi playfully got a little upset and said, 'Aunty, please go away now, I will take care of feeding Kittu'.

After having breakfast she started asking questions from the entire book and he answered every question correctly. **Both of them** had **eaten** fish curry and rice in the afternoon and then Nidhi stopped asking questions and started giving mathematics questions. This continued till 11 o'clock in the night but as it was already night, she had to go home. After she left, his mother settled into a nearby mat, exhaustion a heavy weight on her shoulders after a long day of caring for her son. In the soft glow of the dimly lit room, Kittu continued to immerse himself in the pages of his book, his mother occasionally offering him bites of food to keep his mind and body nourished. With gentle words of encouragement, she urged him along, her love and support acting as a comforting presence by his side.

As Kittu turned each page, his determination grew, spurred on by the promise written within the book that success awaited those who diligently pursued their studies.

He focused intently on the text before him, absorbing every word with unwavering concentration. The weight of the upcoming entrance examination hung in the air, a challenge that both excited and intimidated him in equal measure.

With each passing moment, Kittu inched closer to the designated page that held the key to his success. His mother observed his dedicated efforts, a sense of pride swelling in her chest as she witnessed her son's tenacity and perseverance. And then, finally, he reached that pivotal moment in the book, the page that held the promise of triumph for those who had come this far.

As the words on the page seeped into his mind, exhaustion crept upon him like a heavy blanket, pulling at his eyelids and beckoning him to rest.

The weariness of the day weighed heavily on his young shoulders, and soon, the comforting embrace of slumber enveloped him as he drifted off to sleep.

His mother, ever vigilant and caring, noticed his descent into sleep and rose from her mat with a tender smile. Gently lifting her son into her arms, she carried him to his bed, tucking him in with a mother's touch that exuded warmth and love. As Kittu settled into a peaceful sleep, his mother brushed a soft kiss upon his forehead, a silent gesture of affection that spoke volumes of her unwavering devotion to her child.

In the quiet of the room, mother and son found solace in the restful embrace of sleep, their intertwined dreams weaving a tapestry of love and familial bond. Despite the challenges and fatigue that marked their daily lives, their shared moments of tenderness and care illuminated the profound connection that bound them together, a bond that transcended words and actions.

And so, in the hush of the night, mother and son found respite in each other's presence, a silent promise of unwavering support and love that would guide them through the trials and triumphs that lay ahead. As sleep claimed them both, their intertwined spirits danced in the realm of dreams, united in a bond that nothing could sever.

Examination day ,end of waiting for JNV exam

.12th February – A new morning, ready to write a new story, ready to roar in the whole world, breaking the shackles of poverty and coming out of problems.

" Without slippers on my feet, without proper clothes on my body, I am coming. Write your destiny with your own hands."

Papa, Mummy, and Nidhi all three went to Lord Shiva's temple together at 5 a.m. In the morning. They all came back by 6:30 a.m.! Mrs. J applied tilak to Kittu and gave him Prasad to eat. He continued his studies. Then, after some time, his father said, 'Son, there might be traffic, so we would leave 1 hour earlier.' Kittu said, 'Ok, father. 'The exam began at 10:30 AM, with entry required by 10 AM.

At 8:30 AM, Mummy fed curd to Kittu. Kittu touched Papa's and Mummy's feet for blessings. He then sat in the rickshaw. Both Mother and Nidhi wished Kittu good luck before Mr. J took his son to the examination centre.

Mr. J reached R. Mitra school (examination centre) by 9:30 a.m. When Kittu got down from the rickshaw, his father said that it would be great to give the exam well and not get nervous. Kittu nodded, said yes, took blessings from Papa, and went inside the school. After entering, he met a teacher who told him in which classroom his exam would be held. He went to the classroom as instructed by the teacher. Inside the examination hall, almost all the children of his school were in the same classroom where Kittu's exam was taking place. There was a lot of noise because all the children were from government schools, so nobody knew anything about discipline. Two teachers were in the classroom, one of whom got angry and started slapping the children. Kittu also got slapped and became very scared. After the beating, all the students in the class became completely silent. The students got the question paper at 10:15 AM, along with an OMR sheet. It was said that everyone would first fill in their name on the OMR sheet and then read the questions. No one should attempt the questions before 10:30 AM; they should only read quickly. When the bell rings, everyone can start solving the questions. Some children did not know how to fill out the OMR, so the teacher explained to all the students how to fill out the OMR well. At precisely 10:30 AM, the sound of the bell echoed through the examination hall, signalling the commencement of the questioning session. The teacher, with authoritative poise, directed the eager students to begin formulating their inquiries. With a warm encouragement, the teacher wished all the students the best before settling into a watchful vigil over the examination proceedings.

As the examination progressed, the invigilator maintained a watchful eye over the students. A few individuals, unable to resist the temptation of distractions, found themselves cautioned by the vigilant invigilator.

Amidst the tension of the examination environment, a curious incident unfolded. A girl positioned behind Kittu was observed replicating his every move. It appeared that Kittu, inadvertently or otherwise, was unknowingly aiding the girl in her endeavour. The similarity of the questions misled the young accomplices, as the cunning difference in question numbering went unnoticed, leading to a potentially compromising situation.

Such instances serve as a reminder of the importance of integrity in academic settings, and the necessity of upholding the principles of honesty and fair play.

1:15 PM: There were some questions left in the Hindi paragraph, so he solved whatever he felt was right by remembering the name of God and mother.

1:30 PM: Invigilator took the question paper along with the OMR. Kittu started coming out of the examination room. For the first time in his life, he had seen such a huge crowd of students. All were leaving the examination centre. As soon as he came out, he saw a very strange scene. It was also the first time in his life that the parents of the children were standing in two queues, and the children were walking through the middle of those queues. Poor Kittu's eyes were searching for his father in both rows. He could not see where his father was standing. He was going ahead when a voice came from behind, Kittu. When he turned and looked, the voice was that of his father.

His father picked him up in his lap and asked him, 'Son, how did you do in the exam?' Kittu said, 'papa, excellent.' Hearing this, his eyes became moist and he congratulated his son. Then they made him sit on the rickshaw and took him home.

As soon as they both reached home, Mrs. J and Nidhi said to Kittu: 'We know that your exam went very, very well.' Hearing this, a smile appeared on his face and he said to his mother, 'Mom, don't worry, whatever you think, I will do everything.' Hearing this, Mrs. J's eyes filled with tears and she hugged Kittu to her chest and blessed him.

In the evening, an uncle came to meet Kittu and said to him 'Son, I forgot to mention that there is also negative marking.' Kittu did not know anything about it, nor did he understand; he just smiled after listening to the uncle.

Mr. J and Mrs. J were discussing late at night, and Mr. J mentioned that someone brought a bike or a big vehicle to the exam centre. He also noticed that the parents of the other children appeared to be well-educated. How will our child succeed in the exam among students with such advantages? It's concerning that our child doesn't receive good tuition or sufficient teaching from us to compete effectively.

Hearing all these things, Mrs. J replied, 'Even if we are not able to give good tuition, even if we are not educated, even if we do not have a car or money, our deeds are good and our good deeds alone are enough to give success to our son. Whatever source our son got to read, he read it thoroughly and God is witness to everything; our son will definitely get success.'

Upon hearing all this, Mr. J felt satisfied and a little better, but both were still worried.

13th February: Mr. J **was** told by his neighbours that something ha**d** gone wrong in the JNV entrance exam and the exam w**ould** be held again. Mr. J g**ot** nervous because of this and he immediately **went** home and **told** Kittu about this. Kittu **said**: 'Papa, don't worry. I w**ould** go to school tomorrow and find out.'

On 14th February at 10:20am,

Kittu asked, 'Sir, Sir, will the JNV entrance exam be held again?'

Sir said, 'No, child. It will happen at one or two places. Don't worry, it won't be yours.'

He wanted to tell this to his father quickly because his father was very worried about this. But he was about to leave at 4 o'clock and he did not want to wait until evening. He gave the school bag to one of his friends and asked him to deliver it to his home in the evening. Then he came home, but his father was not there.

At 1:00 PM, the weather was chilly, yet Mr. J appeared utterly soaked in sweat, resembling someone who had just emerged from a bath. He had arrived home to have a meal. Observing Papa's exhausted state, Kittu felt a pang of concern. Papa proceeded to refresh himself by splashing water on his face and feet before inquiring why Kittu had returned from school earlier than usual. With a sense of urgency, Kittu relayed, "Papa, concerning your worry about my exam possibly being repeated, I wanted to reassure you that it **would** not occur. Errors **might** had transpired in certain places. I needed to inform you promptly, hence my early return." The poignant interaction between father and son conveyed a sense of familial devotion and responsibility.

Mr. J became completely calm after listening to his son's words and did not say anything for some time. He was thinking that his son **was** so young and already thinks so much about his parents. His eyes became moist, and he made him sit on his lap and started feeding him with his hands. Seeing this scene, Mrs. J felt very happy.

Worried about Nidhi's absence, Kittu was enjoying his favourite foods, gram, and puri prepared at night.

After the meal, as everyone settled to sleep, Kittu suddenly questioned his mother about Nidhi's whereabouts. His mother was clueless and advised him to ask his father. Upon asking his father, Kittu learned that Nidhi had left Deoghar. Immediately, he inquired, 'Papa, when would they all come?' to which his father sadly replied, 'Son, they had left Deoghar and wouldl not return.'

His heart sank upon knowing that Nidhi would not be coming back, leaving him feeling very uneasy and anxious. Subsequently, he quietly went to his mother and sought solace by sleeping beside her.

Next morning,

Mrs. J. Nandlal, wake up. Won't you go to school? Wake up, son!

Kittu: I won't go, mother. I don't feel like going today. (He was very sad because of Nidhi).

Mrs. J: You get up after some time, brush your teeth, and eat something.

Kittu: Mother, where are you going?

Mrs. J: Going to bring cow dung.

Kittu: I will also go.

Mrs. J: Son, you study. I will do all this.

Kittu: No, Mom. I also want to go. Kittu stubbornly went with his mother.

Mrs. J kept a basket on her head, and Kittu also kept a small basket on his head. Both of them went to get cow dung. When they had gone some distance from the house (Motka Badiyan) and saw some cow dung there, Kittu said, 'Maa, first I would fill my basket, and then you filled yours.' He started picking up dung with his soft hands, filling it in the basket with one hand, and pressing his nose with the other hand. Seeing this, his mother started laughing loudly. Then both of them went further, and both of their baskets were filled. After both the baskets were filled, they came home.

After coming home, Kittu started cleaning the house. He swept the entire house and courtyard while his mother started cooking. After sweeping and mopping, he also helped in cooking. Mrs. J cooked in an earthen stove, so she had to put wood in it. The better the wood burns, the less smoke will be released.

If the fire went out, it had to be lit by blowing air through the mouth. Today Kittu also did all this work.

When he was helping his mother in cooking, a question came to his mind and he asked his mother: 'When will we cook food with gas?'

His mother replied very lovingly, 'Son, when you complete your studies and get a government job, then we will cook food with gas.'

Together, they prepared potatoes and rice for lunch, and Dal was rarely cooked in their house. But still, they were very happy to eat it. In the afternoon, Mr. And Mrs. J and Kittu had lunch with great pleasure, and the rest of the brothers and sisters went to school. After eating, Mr. J rested for some time and then went to work, while Mrs. J was removing lice from the head of her beloved Nandlal. While doing all this, it became evening, and now Mrs. J had to go cut wood for cooking. Kittu also started insisting that he would also go with them, and he did.

Tarni Ahra (where they went to cut wood); Both Mrs. J and Kittu were cutting wood. They were also cutting the wood and keeping it in one place. Kittu was just a small boy so he was not able to cut it properly; thus, he would cut one or two with difficulty, while the rest he was picking up the wood cut by his mother and keeping it at his place, to show that he had cut all this. There were many mosquitoes , biting everywhere on hands, feet, and mouth.

A lot of wood had been cut, and the dark shadow of the night had also started covering the evening light.

Mrs. J started preparing to carry the wood. She took two thin ropes, but they were very strong. She spread those ropes on the ground and started placing wood on them. Then, after placing all the wood, she started tying it. While she was tying, Kittu started screaming and said that he too had been bitten. 'Tie it, I would also carry the wood on my head and take it home,' then his mother explained that he was a child. How would he carry it? But he did not agree, so some wood had to be tied for him too.

After tying the woods, both of them placed the bundles on their heads and started walking towards home. By the time they reached home, it was completely dark. When they both had reached near the house, some neighbours were making fun of them for bringing wood. Mrs. J ignored all these comments, but Kittu was getting very angry and asked his mom, 'were we stealing or doing something wrong? My father had no money, that's why **we** couldn't cook with gas. Why were they all saying this?' He was completely irritated.

Then his mother explained to him that those who become very successful in their life, Babu, everyone first makes fun of them. And when they become successful, the same people who made fun of them praise them a lot. Mrs. J asked her Nandlal to make a promise that whenever anyone speaks such words or tries to tease or humiliate them, they should smile instead of getting irritated. Kittu promises that from now on, if anyone would says insulting things, he would smile.

While both of them were talking, they did not realize when they reached home. After reaching home, both of them took a bath and offered evening incense sticks. Kittu was very tired, so he laid down on the bed to rest, and his mother again got busy with her work. While he was resting, he started missing Nidhi a lot but what else could he do other than think.

At night time, after dinner, Mrs. J was massaging Mr. J's feet. While massaging his feet, she told her husband about all the work that Kittu had done during the day. Mr. J became very emotional after hearing all this and told Mrs. J to stop massaging his feet and come sit next to him. Mrs. J sits next to her husband.

Encouragingly, Mr. J began speaking right after she sat next to him, expressing his pride in their son's dedication to his studies and his devotion to serving his parents. He believed that Kittu would attain great success in life and will become a source of inspiration for the less fortunate, ultimately bringing honour to the entire community.

Annual examination

March 1st: In the evening, sitting in his mother's lap, Kittu was saying that his annual examination was going to start from 2nd March.

Mrs J: Son, your preparation must have been complete, I already know it.

Kittu: I have done all the preparation, but the exam is not conducted properly; almost all the children in the class copy each other.

Mrs J: Son, you should not do this. If other students do it, then explain to them also that those who do such things join the crowd of dirty children, and it does not suit the one who wants to move ahead of the crowd, who wants to do something great in life.

Kittu, I neither used to copy, nor do I do, nor will I do so, and I will advise others not to copy either.

Mrs. J, well done my dear son.

On 2nd March, Thursday, one had to bring the paper from home in order to take the exam. The question paper was not available; the questions were written on the blackboard, and the children wrote their answers on the pages they brought from home.

Kittu took two pages from his brother's new notebook and also took a new pen. After having breakfast, dad had went to work **so he greeted mom only** and then went to school with his elder brother.

At 10:00 a.m., a teacher came to the classroom, wrote questions on the blackboard, and all the children started copying each other and writing answers. It did not seem as if an examination was being conducted in the classroom.

After the exam was over, Kittu ran to his brother and told him that he wanted to eat Pani Puri. The poor guy didn't have any money, so he took 2 rupees from one of his friends and took Kittu to feed him Pani Puri.

Upon reaching the cart, his brother said that he would not eat because 2 rupees were not sufficient, and he wanted to feed only his younger brother.

Kittu did not want to eat alone, so he said that both of them would eat half each, otherwise he wouldn't eat. As a result, they had to eat. After eating Pani Puri, Kittu asked the Pani Puri seller for sour water with tamarind to drink and enjoyed it very much.

By the 5th of March, the examinations were over, and from the next week, Kittu was going to study in 6th grade. It was a very strange thing that without the results of the annual examination, all the students were passed, and the studies of the next class were started.

Even after the exams were over, there were no holidays in the school, nor were there any holidays in the summers, only in the month of July because of the Shravani Mela,which **was** considered to be the longest fair in the world. In this fair, people from all over India came to worship Baba Baidyanath Dham. When there was a huge crowd, Jharkhand Police used to call CRPF, Rapid Action Force, and National Disaster Response Force to control the crowd. All these officers used to stay in government schools.

That is why instead of giving summer leave, leave was given for Shravani Mela.

One day, some people had come to school and they were talking about JNV. So, Kittu thought that perhaps they had come to announce the results of JNV. He ran and went to them, but after reaching there, he came to know that they all had come to sell books for JNV preparation. Knowing this, Kittu became very sad and started wondering when the JNV results would come. Now, even April was over. Thinking about all this, he was feeling uneasy.

The month of May had arrived, and power cuts had also started. There was no electricity in the houses for a long hours because preparations for the Shravani Mela started from May itself. The electricity supply of the entire area was being rectified, due to which electricity was cut. The entire Deoghar was decorated like a newlywed bride. From Sultanganj to Baba Mandir, all kinds of services were provided to Kanwariyas. Thousands of new shops were opened such as tea stalls, food vendors, hotels, tattoo shops, and many beggars also used to come there.

It was said that beggars earned more money than shopkeepers by begging, and this saying was also true to some extent.

Before the beginning of the month of July, the entire Deoghar begins to look like a newly hitched bride. Fine sand was spread on the entire 100 km route so that the feet of all the **Kanwariyas** did not get harmed. They all used to come on empty feet. They used to bring the holy Ganga water from Sultanganj, and that holy water was used to pour on the Shivling at Baba Dham. They used to come from that distance on foot.

On July 2nd, before every Shravani Mela, there was a puja called Dubey Baba Puja where a billy goat was sacrificed. On Sundays, there used to be a market in Rikhiya where peasant's came to sell cows, goats, vegetables, fruits, etc. But most of them went to **sell** goats. Today, Kittu's father and Mr. J's uncle bought a buck. Due to poverty, Mr. J was not able to buy a goat alone, so he used to buy it with his uncle and split it in half.

Dubey Baba Puja#

On 5th July, today there was a puja at Kittu's house. During every Dubey Baba puja, it used to rain heavily, and wherever they all went to perform the puja, there used to be mud. Everyone used to enjoy a lot by worshiping in the rain, and a fair was also organized, bringing a different joy to the fair in the rain.

In the afternoon Mr J and his uncle went for puja and returned by evening. Mrs J and Kittu stayed at home as it was raining heavily so it was not safe to go out. When they all returned after performing the puja, the goat was divided in half. When all this was happening, some thoughts were coming in Kittu's mind…

On July 10, police were deployed at every intersection in Deoghar. A barrier had been erected next to Kittu's house to keep the crowd under control, and holidays had been declared in schools.

First day of Shravani Mela

On 12th July, 'Bol Bam, Bol Bam, Baba Nagari dur hai jana jarur hai, Bhole Baba Patthar Me,Parvati k chakkar me', the entire Deoghar echoed with such slogans. The auspicious start of the Shravani fair has begun today. The Kanwariyas were being welcomed very beautifully by the raindrops, the weather was completely favourable, and all the devotees were in a frenzy in Bhole Baba's city. It seemed that all the devotees had seen Lord Shiva and all the devotees are going crazy with happiness.

On the streets, small children from poor families were begging from kanwariyas. 'Give me one rupee, I am eating biscuits,' someone used to say. Another would claim their mother is unwell. Beggars used to sit on the streets and ask for money in the name of God.

The slogans of Lord Shiva, the voices of children, and the drizzling drops of rain all together enhanced the beauty of the land of Gods. The entire Deoghar was abuzz with joy.

At night, Kittu was saying to his mother, 'Mom, please make a small cloth bag (Battu) for me in which I could keep the money after begging.'

Great day for Mr. J's family

On 13 July, Mrs. J opened her tea stall. Some Bol Bam were drinking tea at the stall, and some were waiting for the tea to be made. Mrs. J was making tea while Kittu was washing the tea glasses behind the shop. Then a boy came to Mrs. J and told her that the JNV results had come and he had to go to the post office to see them. He asked where Kittu was and mentioned that he would go with him. Mrs. J became completely restless, left everything, called Kittu, and told him to stop washing the glasses and go with his friend to see his results. He asked which results, and his mother said, the result of JNV entrance exam.

He felt completely nervous and happy at the same time.

Kittu quickly washed his hands and wiped them on his mother's saree, then sat on Neeraj's bicycle. There was a lot of crowd due to the Shravani Mela all the way. When they reached the post office, they immediately got off the bicycle and went inside. There was an employee, so Kittu asked him if he wanted to see the JNV result. The employee told him to check the list on the wall. They both started searching for their names in the lists. Kittu was completely upset as he could not find his name and was drenched in sweat.

Neeraj instructed Kittu to raise his gaze slightly. Due to his short stature, Kittu was unable to discern the names written above. Upon following Neeraj's advice and looking upwards, Kittu discovered his own name on the list – Kittu Kumar!

To be continued in next part……

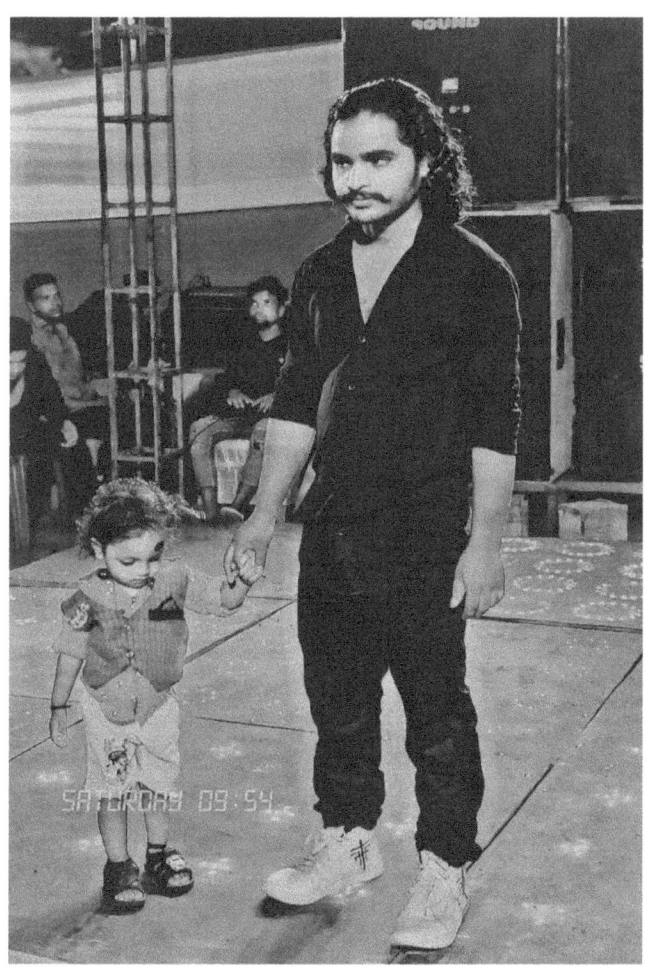

Although every war carries inherent risks, it may not always result in detrimental outcomes.

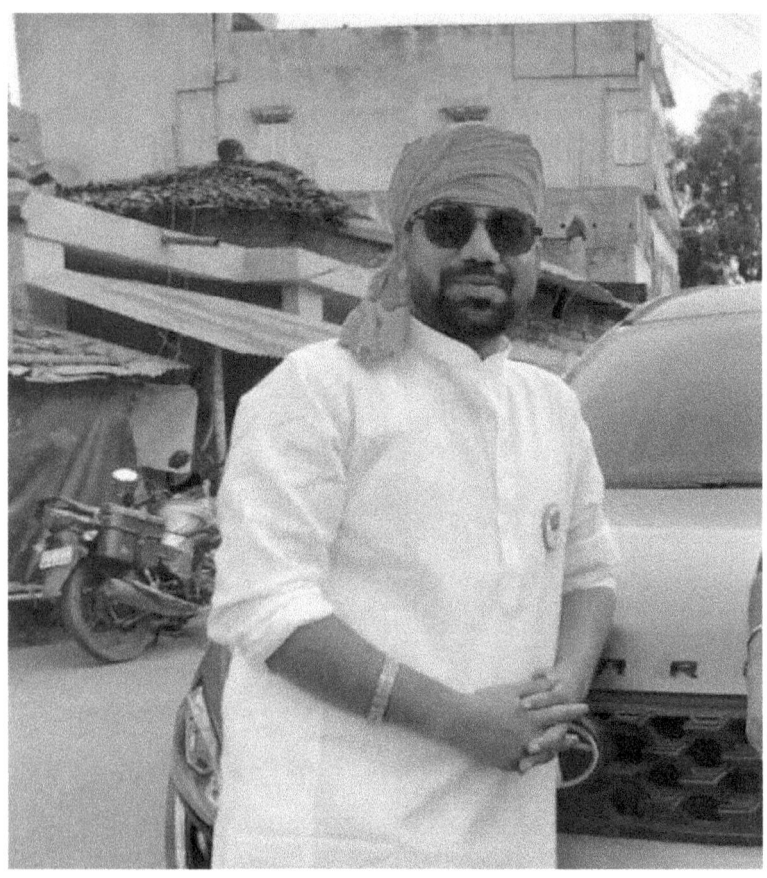

Those who roamed the streets started roaming in safari; those who never took responsibility of the house started taking care of the entire country.

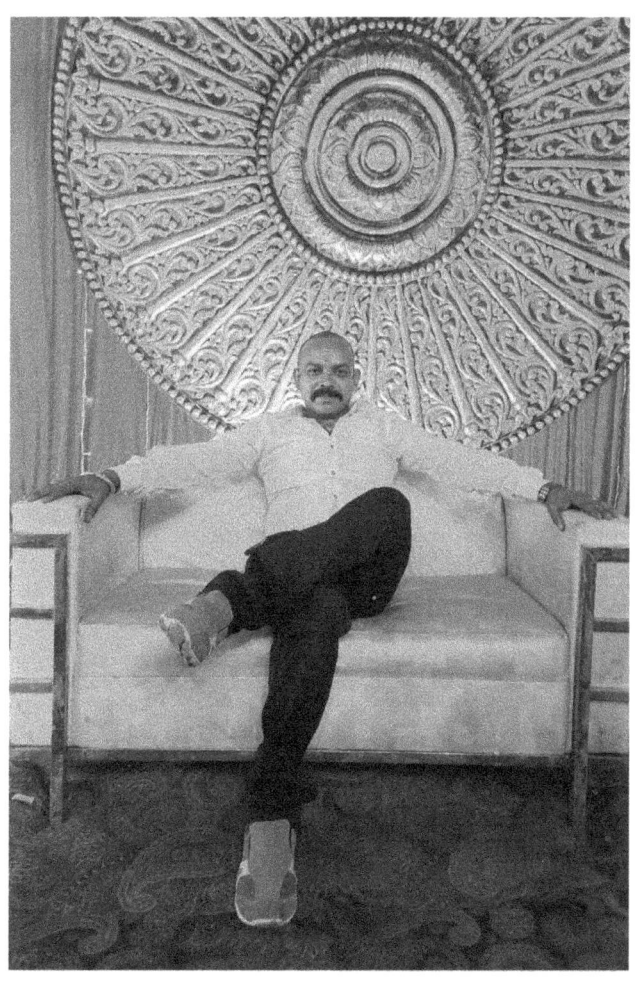

Those individuals whom society once deemed as slaves are now the ones exerting control and dominance over the world.

www.ingramcontent.com/pod-product-compliance
Lightning Source LLC
LaVergne TN
LVHW061602070526
838199LV00077B/7144